The Basics of Kettlebell Exercises

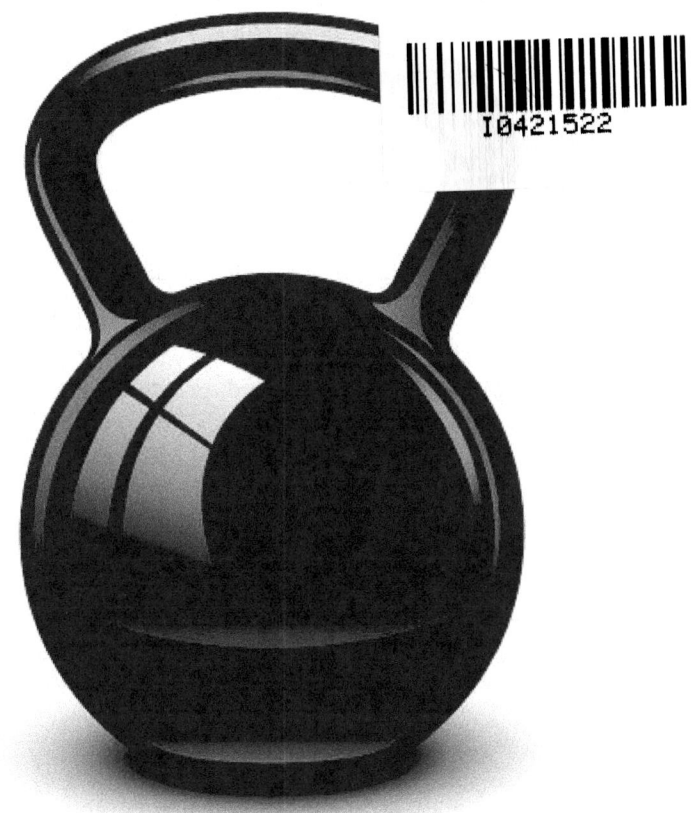

Health Learning Series

M. Usman

Mendon Cottage Books

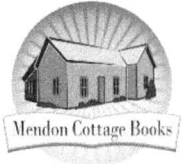

JD-Biz Publishing

Disclaimer

The information is this book is provided for informational purposes only. It is not intended to be used and medical advice or a substitute for proper medical treatment by a qualified health care provider. The information is believed to be accurate as presented based on research by the author.

The contents have not been evaluated by the U.S. Food and Drug Administration or any other Government or Health Organization and the contents in this book are not to be used to treat cure or prevent disease.

The author or publisher is not responsible for the use or safety of any diet, procedure, or treatment mentioned in this book. The author or publisher is not responsible for errors or omissions that may exist.

Warning

The Book is for informational purposes only and before taking on any diet, treatment, or medical procedure, it is recommended to consult with your primary health care provider.

Our books are available at

1. Amazon.com
2. Barnes and Noble
3. Itunes
4. Kobo
5. Smashwords
6. Google Play Books

Table of Contents

Introduction

In addition to being a fitness tool, the kettlebell has now become a very famous form of showmanship. It's a well-known fact that kettlebells pack a plethora of health benefits, but nowadays, kettlebells are becoming increasingly popular among sportsmen, fighters, wrestlers due to the countless muscular benefits they pack. Kettlebells offer one of the easiest and most affordable types of workout, and a large number of fitness experts and professionals are working on kettlebells, which makes the entire help and support process so much easier.

This type of workout can be performed quite easily, as it does not require any kind of extra efforts to be put in. All you need is a medium sized kettlebell, some free space to workout in your home, and a firm concept about what you are going to do.

If you want to know the basics about how kettlebell workouts operate and how you can be able to perform various workouts for getting ultimate health benefits, then you can take the advantage of this book, which will answer each and every query you have about the sport.

You can take several actions while working with kettlebells, including pressing, floor pressing, overhead squats and rows, etc. All these postures will definitely help you out in getting what you want to achieve by making you able to practice all the types of workouts easily. In this book you will find all the ways by which you can do the workout without any problem.

Not only this, but after going through this book, you will get to know the ultimate health benefits and the proven steps for getting the ultimate fat burning out of your body by doing some simple kettlebell workouts.

This book will definitely help you in getting all the answers related to kettlebell workouts and the benefits related to it.

Getting Started

Chapter # 1: Know about kettlebell exercises

Kettlebell workouts are known to be some of the most mysterious workouts, as they do not require you to put too much effort, especially efforts that go to waste. But, no matter how mysterious it seems to be, it has been gaining popularity and more and more trainers and professionals are providing training for it. This is so the fitness of the people they are training does not come under any sort of compromise.

It doesn't matter if you want to lose excess fats or want to build your body's muscles, the kettlebell workouts will definitely help you in achieving your ultimate goal. Overall it can be said that the kettlebell will grant you so many benefits that no other workout will provide you.

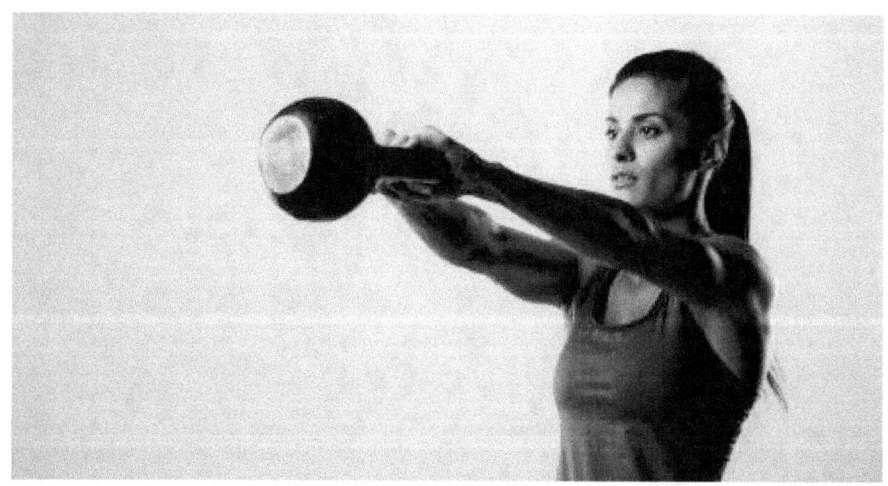

Kettlebell workouts are the most powerful tools through which you'll be able to reach you maximum potential, something that is very tough to accomplish otherwise. All you need is to have full coordination with the various acts of sports or any other act that you want to engage with kettlebell workout. As a result, you will be able to transfer your workout to any of the sports you want.

If you do the kettlebell workouts given in the book, on a regular basis, you will be able to make improvements in your overall cardiovascular health as well. This will lead to improved jumping capability or any springing action that you require in daily life.

The duration for workouts may vary from 4 to 10 weeks depending upon your wish. You can increase or decrease the duration of doing each exercise by what you want. But you should consider that the minimum duration of doing these workouts is 2 weeks or 15 days.

The kettlebell training cycle may vary from person to person, but it is mandatory that you should opt for this workout at least twice a week in the beginning, and then start moving forward by making the duration longer than before.

Chapter # 2: Get the Ultimate Health Benefits

As for my concern, I would say that kettlebell exercises provide you with ultimate health benefits, which no other exercise can provide, in most cases. One of the most significant advantages that it gives you is the extent of its simplicity, as all the workouts done under this type of exercise are very simple. Therefore you don't need any extra effort to be put in other than having a firm grip so that you don't drop the kettle bell on your head!

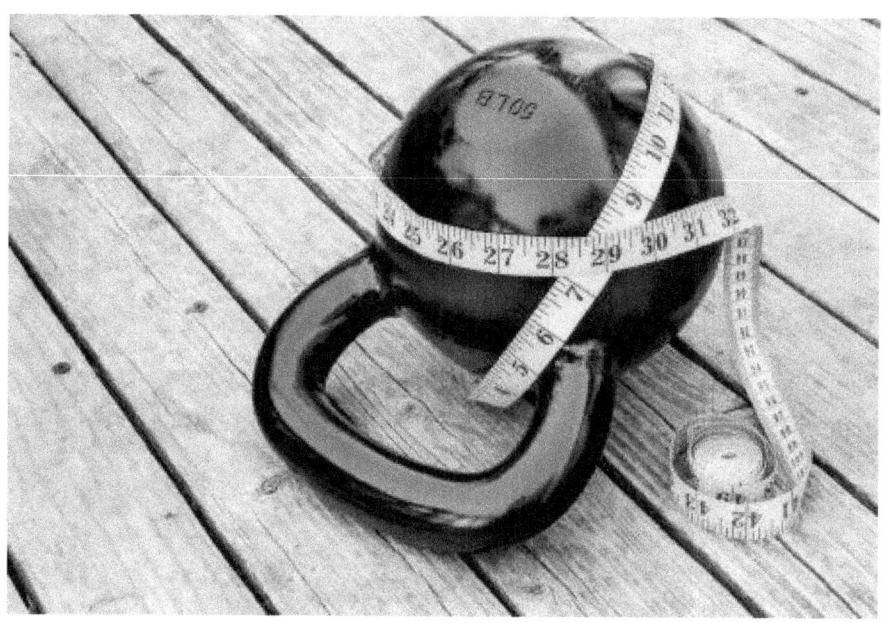

You are not required to invest a large amount of money for getting the kettlebells, as they are very affordable and can be accessed and kept at the place where you work/study without any problem. You should not face any sort of problem while moving them from one place to another and they can be stored anywhere due to their size. An additional characteristic that they possess is they are not as ugly as dumbbells and thus you will not feel any kind of awkwardness while using them.

Here are a few benefits you can reap if you use kettlebells during workouts, as given in the book.

Offsetting of center of gravity

The offsetting of the center of gravity is done by using the kettlebells, which maximizes the strength imparted to the shoulders and overall health. Not just this, but they also help in bringing much needed flexibility to the body. These kettlebells not only prevent joint injuries, but also proactively improve the joints' current stature.

Imparting strength to lower back

While you work with kettlebells, they will help you in getting the ultimate strength and grip to the lower part of your back and also help in giving strength to your back. Additionally, they will help you a lot in gaining flexibility with the help of swings, which you perform while doing the kettlebell workouts.

Making the workouts easy

If you are dealing with some workouts that are of high intensity then kettlebells will help you out in making those workouts extremely easy and you can go through them without any problem.

Get the ultimate simplicity

You can work with so much simplicity with the kettlebell workouts that you will not face any sort of issues. You will get the freedom of working out easily with them and there are very simple workout procedures are available. You can make your own workout plan very effortlessly and you can benefit from the highest level of workouts.

Forget the gym

One of the biggest benefits that kettlebell workouts grant you is that if you work with it as you should, by following all the instructions, and then you will be able to have your own workout sessions at your home. Then, you can get rid of your heavy and hectic routine associated with gym. So, you do not need to go to gym when you are working out with kettlebells at your home.

Varieties of Kettlebell Exercises

Chapter # 1: Introduction

Right now, you think that you have to go to a gym for an intense workout for ultimate body strength. But with kettlebells, you do not need to opt for the gym, as you will get all the health benefits at your home with the help of these user-friendly workouts which you will love. Each and every muscle of your body can be targeted using these workouts, and you will be able to give your muscles the ultimate strength that not even dumbbells can grant you.

The kettlebells are proven to be an effective tool to impart ultimate strength to your body, and, in the bodybuilding act of Russia, these workouts work as a primary tool for getting the desired results. Not only is this true, but the strongest man in Russia is often called the man of kettle bells.

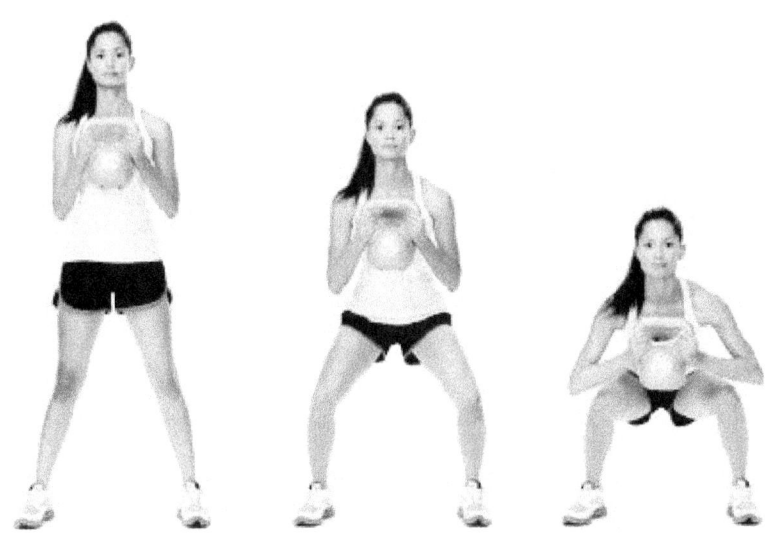

Various types of kettlebell workouts are there and they vary from one person to another depending upon the will of the person who is going to perform it. Some people enjoy each and every workout that is associated with kettlebells, as they continue with a form of training that is resistive in nature. This helps them in getting the desired results that they want. For continuing with this type of training, relatively higher weights are used, which help the trainer in getting what he actually wants related to his bodily health.

There are certain people, as well, who opt for working out with kettlebells owing to the fact that they want a complete body cardio circuit. This type of working out uses relatively lighter weights and is used by the trainers, followed by the repetition of each and every act they do for making their body strong.

No matter whatever type of workout you chose for your body, you will always get a lot of benefits from working with kettlebells. These workouts will not cost you very much at all. All the workouts with kettlebells are truly versatile, and, with just a small amount of equipment, you can get what you want for the strength of your body.

Here, you are going to have some of the kettlebell workouts that you can opt for, according to your wish and desire. All of these varieties will definitely help you out in getting the ultimate health benefits, for sure.

Chapter # 2: Double Kettlebell Squat

Honestly speaking, this type of kettlebell workout would be very easy to explain, but it is a little bit difficult to do. In this type of workout, you need two kettlebells to squat with.

How to do the exercise

All you need to do is hold the kettlebells in front of both of your shoulders. If you think that it is somehow difficult, then you can opt for taking them in both of your hands first, and then move the hands upwards till shoulders' height to get in the correct position.

➤ Now you are required to squat as low as you can and here your knees will also come into action.

➤ While doing this, instead of getting your knees straight on the floor, you have to keep your knees on the outer sides.

➤ In this posture, your spine should be exactly straight and it must be stacked upon your pelvis area.

➤ The act which you are required to do here is to not let your shoulders slump in the forward direction, in any case.

➤ Now you must be in a standing posture while keeping the back straight, and then you are required to repeat the same process.

Chapter # 3: Turkish Get Up

This type of workout will not only help you in bringing strength to your body, but will also help you in making corrections to the muscles which have become imbalanced for any reason. This type of kettlebell workout should be a part of your regular routine so that you can become able to get the desired results related to your health.

How to do the exercise

➢ At the initial stage, lie down on the floor and make sure your right arm is extended straight, in such a way that it may come in front of your chest. Your shoulders in this posture should be down.

➢ Your back should remain straight and flat on the ground. Now it's time to make a bend in your right knee.

➢ Put all your weight on the left elbow and try to get into the sitting position.

➢ Now, sit up straight while you are going to raise the kettlebell in the direction that leads it over your head.

➢ Repeat this process and then do the following steps:

➢ After you have done this, your right foot must be on the ground flat. Now, it's time to get pushed up by taking strength from your left elbow, followed by making your arm straight in the forward direction.

➢ At the same time, you are going to lift up your chest in the upward direction.

- When you are shifting from one position to the next, your eyes should be on the weight you are carrying with you.

- Your next focus should be your hips, which you are going to lift just after going through the above-mentioned step.

- While you are lifting up the hips, your feet must be flat on the ground and you are not required to lift your feet in this posture. Keep the hips apart from each other at a certain distance.

- Now you have to be in the kneeling position for which you have to take your left leg behind your back.

- While you are doing this, you will notice that you have your right arm still in the extension form above your head.

- Now it's time to stand up in the same posture by putting the left knee from the ground. Now you are done.

- Repeat this process and surely you will go through it very easily without any problem.

Chapter # 4: Kettlebell Pushup Plus

If you want to make the pushups of your daily routine difficult, then the best way by which you can achieve this is by keeping the handles of kettlebells in your hand. Start off by grabbing one kettlebell in each hand.

By doing this, you will be able to get a base that is slightly stable and that will allow you to sink down in the motion range lower than before.

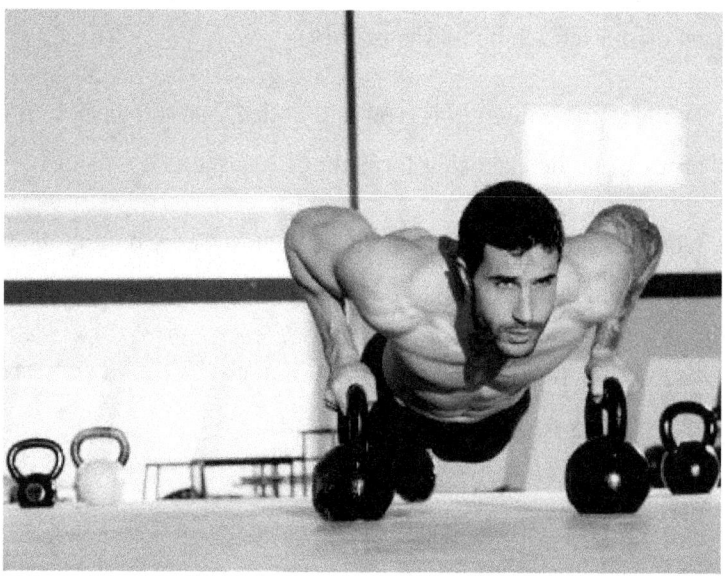

How to do this exercise

If you are looking at taking this step to a higher level, then you should follow the below mentioned steps:

➢ Start by flipping both of the kettlebells over and rest your hands on the bottom side.

➤ After doing this, and when you become successful in keeping the handle in balance with your hand, you will be able to increase the amount of stability.

➤ If the above-mentioned posture seems to be stable for you, then you can give a try to tap your shoulders to the handles. While doing so, the level of your hips should be normal and straight followed by the lighting up of your right hand in the direction close to the left shoulder.

➤ Do not twist your body in any case and repeat the above process as per your requirements.

Chapter # 5: Russian Kettlebell Twist

The Russian kettlebell twist is a fairly simply exercise that can be executed without much hassle. Its steps are as follows:

➤ Assume the sit-up position and place a kettlebell on either one of your sides.

➤ Slightly bend your legs.

➤ Pick up the kettlebell that rests on your side and move it all the way to the opposite side in a controlled, twisting motion.

➤ Twist your back as much as you can without overextending.

Remember, you must always have control over the kettlebell and your body throughout the movement.

Workout for Burning Fat

Chapter # 1: Introduction

People looking to lose weight through kettlebell exercises can follow this workout. It uses a low weight, high reps technique to not just shave off fat, but tone muscle content.

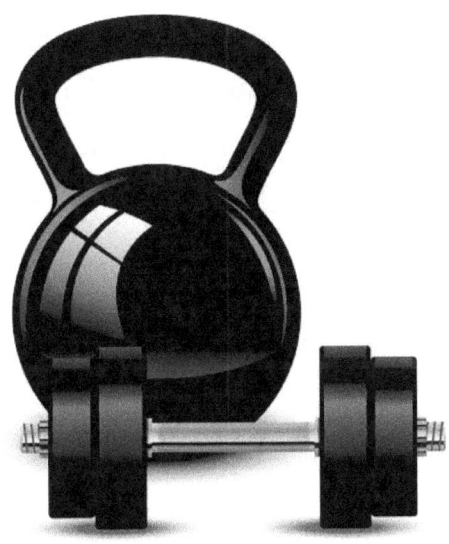

The purpose of kettlebells is to engage the entire body in a workout. So the workout that I'm about to describe will ensure that all parts of the body lose extra weight. In addition, the workout will be perfect for those who have a tough schedule.

Tools Required:

You will need the following equipment for starting the workout:

Men: 35 lbs (16 kg) pair of kettlebells

Women: 18 lbs (8 kg) pair of kettlebells

You will also need a medicine ball that should be 10 lbs (5kg) in weight or equivalent weight plates.

Finally, you'll need an open space that is free of any delicate materials that may get damaged if you drop the kettlebell by accident.

Directions:

The circuit given in the subsequent chapters must be repeated 4–5 times a week. Definitely do not go below twice a week under any circumstance. The directions for each of the exercises are given in the chapters below.

Chapter # 2: Double Handed Kettlebell Swing

Reps: 15

The kettlebell swing is the backbone of the entire Kettlebell workout. Whether it's one dedicated to gain strength or lose weight, it makes up for an energetic, exhilarating workout. This is why it's one of the first workouts anyone learns to perform. Kettlebell swings are easy to learn and help develop a strong posture, the glutes, shoulders, hamstrings, and back.

In a nutshell, the kettlebell swing treats all the muscles that are required in a vertical leap, but, instead of moving into the air, you transfer all your energy into the kettlebell. The kettlebell holds vital importance here, as it improves the work capacity of the person without wasting too much energy on jumping.

The steps are as follows:

1. Assume a wide stance and place your feet almost 1.5–2 times your shoulder width, with toes pointing in the forward direction. The step is vital and you should leave adequate space for the kettlebell, as it will swing in between your legs. The stance will provide you stability and control.

2. Next, squat down, keeping your back straight. This does not mean that you have to keep your back vertical, but keep it slightly arched. Lift up the weight and look across the room as you do so until the squat is complete.

3. To start the movement, squat down and push your hips back until the bell passes your groin. Now, flick the kettlebell back in between your legs and make use of the arms to push the kettlebell across the

line. During the swing, the arms should never be engaged in moving the weight of the kettlebell.

At this stage of the swing, you will have your forearms exerting a force against your groin and the kettlebell extending past you. As the kettlebell reaches its peak decline, execute a squat and begin thrusting your pelvis in the forward direction.

4.   As you squat up, your back will come under strain, which will make the kettlebell propel in the forward direction. Try to propel the kettlebell as far as your chest, but as you do so, you should have complete control over the movement.

In order to repeat the exercise, let the bell fall back into the arc and repeat the movement once again.

Chapter # 3: Clean

Reps: 12–15, each arm

The kettlebell exercise known as clean is performed to learn other complex exercises. However, it does target specific muscle groups, i.e. glutes, core, hamstrings, and lower back. The exercise involves lifting up a kettlebell right in front of the shoulders and resting it on the forearm. The movement is of vital importance in exercises like the front squats and kettlebell press.

The steps are as follows:

1.   Start off in the deadlift position, holding the kettlebell in between your legs. Remember, the clean is a swift movement, like a vertical jump, but instead of jumping you'll be transferring your energy into the kettlebell.

2.   Drive up the kettlebell, keeping your arms bent instead of extending them. This will keep the weight close to the body. The arms should be kept static in the movement, e.g. used like a rope, to carry the weight around.

3.   As soon as the kettlebell reaches your chest, tuck your arms under the bell so that you successfully lock in the kettlebell's position.

4.   By now, you would've reached the final position, known as the racked position or the "Clean" position. Notice you entire body's position, i.e. the straightness of your wrists, the lightness of your forearms, and strain on your upper arms.

Throughout the exercise, you must remain in control of the kettlebell and drop it to the safest point if an emergency pops up.

Chapter # 4: Press

Reps: 12–15, each arm

The kettlebell press in an outstanding exercise aimed to build shoulder strength, in addition to the laterals and biceps. In order to perform the exercise, you need to start off with the rack or clean position.

The steps are as follows:

1.   Starting off in the rack position, make sure that your body is tight, tensed from shoulders down, and elbows in. Throughout the movement, your waist will need to be supported by tightening your ab muscles. Do not, under any circumstance, try to propel the bell in the air using energy derived from your legs.

2.   When in the rack position, rotate your shoulders so that the forearms are straight and the backside of your hand is parallel to your back.

3.   During the kettlebell press, the bell will follow a banana-shaped arc, i.e. it will get lifted outwards and then in an upward direction. As you perform the lift, keep your shoulders strong.

4.   Now, lift the bell straight up until the arm is fully vertical and locked out.

Here are a few tips that will help you during the exercise:

•   When you're in the clean position, lower your shoulders as far down as you can so that the muscles in and around the shoulders are stretched out. This will allow you to load up the muscles and have better leverage.

- At the stretched out position, your elbows should touch the hipbone.

- Bring out your back muscles (laterals) so that they stretch completely outwards. This will bring in much needed stability to the workout.

- Hold the handles of each kettlebell as tightly as possible so that you don't drop them over your head during lifting.

- When lifting the kettlebell, instead of focusing on actually lifting it, focus on resisting moving into the ground.

Note: The next exercise is the Russian Twist which is the same as given in Variety of Kettle bell Exercises: Chapter 5; it requires 8 reps, each side.

Chapter #5: Push-Press

Reps: 12–15, each side

After performing the Russian Twist, move on to the Push-Press which is as follows:

1. Begin the exercise in the push up position, assuming the plank position, facing the floor. Your arms should make a 90 degree angle against the floor, and you should be holding 2 kettlebells, using them to lift yourself.

2. Once you have balanced your weight on top of the kettlebells, perform a push up and bring your chest as close to the ground as possible before pushing away.

3. Once you reach the top position, lift one of the kettlebells off the floor, and balance your entire body's weight on the other. Lift the kettlebell up until your elbows stick out behind your back.

4. Hold the weight for a few seconds, lower it back down, perform anther pushup, and repeat with the other side.

Chapter #6: Single Leg RDL

Reps: 12–15, each side

The exercise is quite simple and the steps are as follows:

1. Stand up straight with your feet shoulder width apart.

2. Pick up the kettlebell with your right hand, and start the movement by lifting your right leg up while simultaneously leaning forward.

3. Maintaining your balance, lower your body as much as you can until the kettlebell just touches the ground.

4. At this point, move in reverse motion until you're in the starting position once again.

Chapter #7: Windmills

Reps: 12–15, each side

This is the final exercise in the workout and it is a fantastic one if you're looking to lose weight and gain oblique strength. The steps are detailed as follows:

1. Start off by standing with your feet at shoulders width. Raise your left hand straight up until it is locked. As soon as the arm is locked, move your hip slightly outwards to increase surface area and thus the balance of your body. Keep your left hand free of any tension and dangling freely.

    During the lift, breathe in and keep the abdominals tight, derive strength from them if you need to.

2. Now, look at the kettlebell and bend the hips towards the right, grazing your right hand all the way down your thigh. As you approach the bottom part of the movement, the leg may start to bend; however, do not force it the other way, as this is completely fine.

3. Continue to slide your right hand down your leg until it touches the feet or the ground. If you do not possess great flexibility, then slide it down as far as possible and don't extend too much or you'll damage your muscles. Don't worry, as you'll build your flexibility with time.

4. Finally, you should be in an almost 90 degree position with both your arms being in a straight line.

During the exercise, if you have to, you should bend a little forward, but never in the backwards direction.

Chapter #8: The Routine

Once you've learned all the exercises, it's time to put them in motion. For that, I've given a brief weekly routine that you should carry out for at least 6 weeks. The tables will help you manage the workout.

During the exercise and when first starting out, aim for a minimal number of reps, so that you don't lose your breath. Rest 1–2 minutes in between each round and don't aim for 6 rounds when starting out, as 3–4 will be fine.

Execute as many rounds as you can in 20 minutes. Before performing any kettlebell exercise, perform 5 minutes of cardio, e.g. treadmill.

Monday's Workout

	Weight	Rd. 1	Rd. 2	Rd. 3	Rd. 4	Rd. 5	Rd. 6
Double kettlebell swing							
Clean							
Press							
Russian twist							
Push press							
Single leg RDL							
Windmills							

Wednesday's Workout

	Weight	Rd. 1	Rd. 2	Rd. 3	Rd. 4	Rd. 5	Rd. 6
Double kettlebell swing							
Clean							
Press							
Russian twist							
Push press							
Single leg RDL							
Windmills							

Friday's Workout

	Weight	Rd. 1	Rd. 2	Rd. 3	Rd. 4	Rd. 5	Rd. 6
Double kettlebell swing							
Clean							
Press							
Russian twist							
Push press							

Single leg RDL							
Windmills							

MMA Workout

Sounds exhilarating, doesn't it?

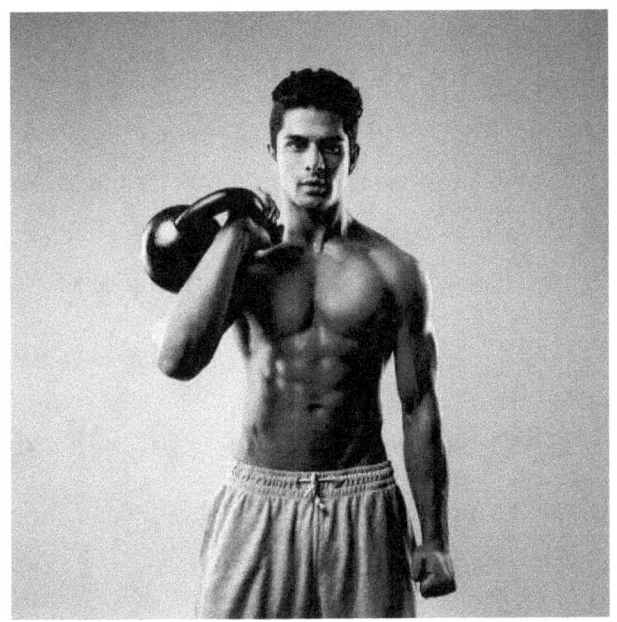

Kettlebell workouts are not just popular among those looking to lose weight, but are also famous among MMA trainers, due to their strength training characteristics. I've given 3 kettlebell exercises that are performed by MMA fighters, and it is recommended that you execute these 3 when you're feeling most energetic. Kettlebell exercises are getting increasingly popular among MMA wrestlers, as they allow the fighter to target various muscle groups more effectively, as compared to the traditional lifting techniques. Without further ado, I present to you the exercises.

Three sets of each of the following exercise would be enough for starters.

Kettlebell Duck Walk – 3x sets, 1 min break:

The exercise's name may sound a little weird but the fact of the matter is that the exercise is widely used by wrestlers across the globe, as it engages and subsequently strengthens the entire body. The exercise works well for both small & large muscles and also improves a fighter's balance.

Start off in a standing position. Take ahold of 2 kettlebells and assume the rack position. Next, clean the bell right up to your shoulder's height while squatting down until the calves make contact with the thighs. Finally, walk up and down like a duck and perform the movement for at least 1 minute. The kettlebell weight should be the same as you would use for swings.

Do not rush the walk, keep your calm, and balance throughout the exercise.

Kettlebell Split Snatch – 3 sets, 5x reps each side:

This exercise requires sheer explosiveness from your body, as it aims to build not only your power, but also the element of surprise in you. The exercise goes as follows:

Start off by holding a kettlebell in between your legs. Squat down keeping your back in an arched position and snatch the kettlebell up. But, here's the tricky part; instead of executing a traditional snatch that involves punching through the zero gravity point, displace your entire body so that the kettlebell moves right over your head.

Keep practicing and you'll surely develop a lot of strength and explosiveness, which will help you execute surprise moves that are essential in wrestling.

Kettlebell Split Jerk – 3x sets, 5x reps each:

The exercise is quite similar to the aforementioned split snatch exercise and uses the same method of moving under the kettlebell.

To execute the exercise, raise the kettlebell into the rack position and then bend your knees. Dip down 2–3 inches, push the kettlebell upwards, and assume the lunge position. Stand up, complete the repetition, and repeat.

The exercise is easier than the split snatch, and if you are unable to execute the split snatch, then you may replace it with this exercise.

Conclusion

That's it from my side. Everything you need to know about kettlebells to gain strength, lose weight, and improve stability has been given in this book. Kettlebells will undoubtedly have a huge positive effect on your health, and will not only help you physically, but will also help you develop greater discipline mentally.

It's up to you now, whether you follow the instructions and reap all the benefits or not. The chapters given in the book are quite comprehensive and provide instructions that can be applied anywhere, at home, or at work. All you need is a pair of kettlebells and you'll be good to go. So, if I were you, I wouldn't wait any longer and dive into the intense, powerful, and disciplined sport of Kettlebell.

Thank you and best of luck!

References

http://www.123rf.com/photo_19314165_kettle-bell-over-white.html

http://www.123rf.com/photo_24747732_young-fitness-female-exercise-with-kettle-bell-mixed-race-woman-doing-crossfit-workout-on-grey-backg.html

http://www.123rf.com/photo_16126200_kettlebell-and-measuring-tape-on-wooden-deck--fitness-and-exercise-concept.html

http://www.123rf.com/photo_13183270_series-of-kettlebell-weight-exercise-sequence-to-promote-strength-and-muscle-tone-please-see-portfol.html

http://www.123rf.com/photo_29223046_portrait-of-strong-young-man-working-out-with-kettle-bell-young-muscular-guy-with-cross-fit-equipmen.html

http://www.123rf.com/photo_17050617_gym-man-push-up-strength-pushup-exercise-with-kettlebell-in-a-crossfit-workout.html

http://www.123rf.com/photo_20228263_kettlebell-and-dumbbell-over-white.html

Author Bio

Muhammad Usman is a distinguished medical graduate of Allama Iqbal medical college (AIMC). He is a professional writer who has been in the field for more than 4 years. During this time he has produced 10,000+ articles, blogs, and eBooks on various niches related to diseases, health, fitness, nutrition, and well-being. He is a regular contributor to several journals related to medicine and surgery. He is the editor of several journals and newspapers.

Check out some of the other JD-Biz Publishing books

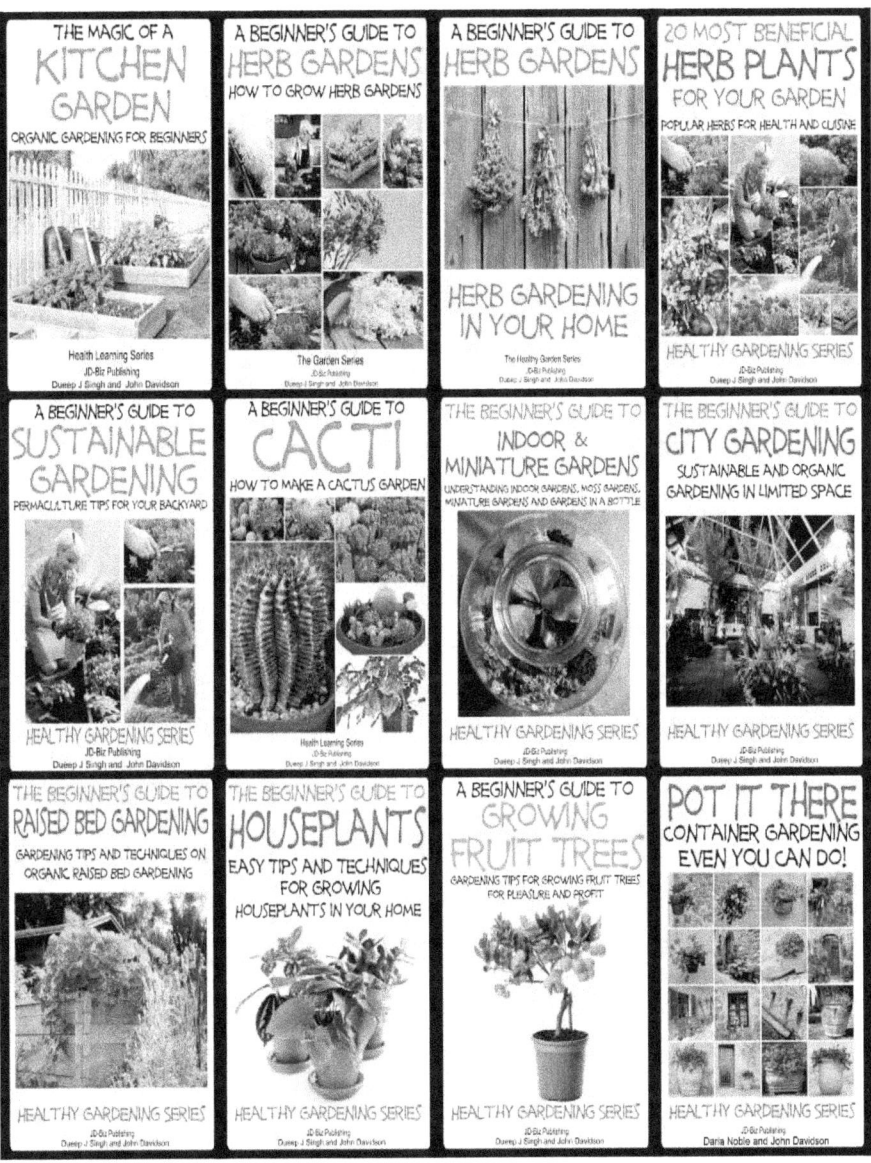

Health Learning Series

THE MAGIC OF GOOSEBERRIES FOR HEALTH AND BEAUTY	THE MAGIC OF YOGURT FOR COOKING AND BEAUTY	THE MAGIC OF LEMONS USING LEMONS FOR HEALTH AND BEAUTY	THE MAGIC OF CHILLIES FOR COOKING AND HEALING	THE MAGIC OF ONIONS ONIONS IN CUISINE TO CURE AND TO HEAL	THE MAGIC OF RADISHES TO CURE AND TO HEAL
THE MAGIC OF CARROTS TO CURE AND TO HEAL	THE MAGIC OF OREGANO FOR COOKING AND HEALTH	THE MAGIC OF MARIGOLDS Marigolds for Health And Beauty	THE HEALTH BENEFITS OF CINNAMON	THE MAGIC OF COCONUTS FOR COOKING & HEALTH	THE MAGIC OF CLOVES FOR HEALING AND COOKING
THE MAGIC OF ASAFETIDA FOR COOKING AND HEALING	THE MAGIC OF NEEM MARGOSA TO HEAL	THE MAGIC OF SALT TO HEAL AND FOR BEAUTY	THE MAGIC OF POMEGRANATES FOR HEALTH AND BEAUTY	THE MAGIC OF DRY FRUIT AND SPICES REMEDIES AND RECIPES	THE HEALTH BENEFITS OF TURMERIC CURCUMIN FOR COOKING AND HEALTH
THE MAGIC OF ALOE VERA	THE MAGIC OF VEGETABLES ANCIENT HEALING REMEDIES AND TIPS	THE HEALTH BENEFITS OF ROSEMARY FOR COOKING AND HEALTH	THE MAGIC OF PEPPER & PEPPERCORNS FOR COOKING & HEALING	THE MAGIC OF MILK, BUTTER AND CHEESE FOR COOKING & HEALING	THE MAGIC OF CARDAMOMS FOR COOKING AND HEALTH
THE HEALTH BENEFITS OF BLACK CUMIN FOR COOKING AND HEALTH	THE MAGIC OF BASIL-TULSI TO HEAL NATURALLY	THE MAGIC OF SPICES FOR HEALTH AND CUISINE	THE MAGIC OF ROSES FOR COOKING AND BEAUTY	The Miraculous Healing Powers of GINGER	The Miracle of HONEY

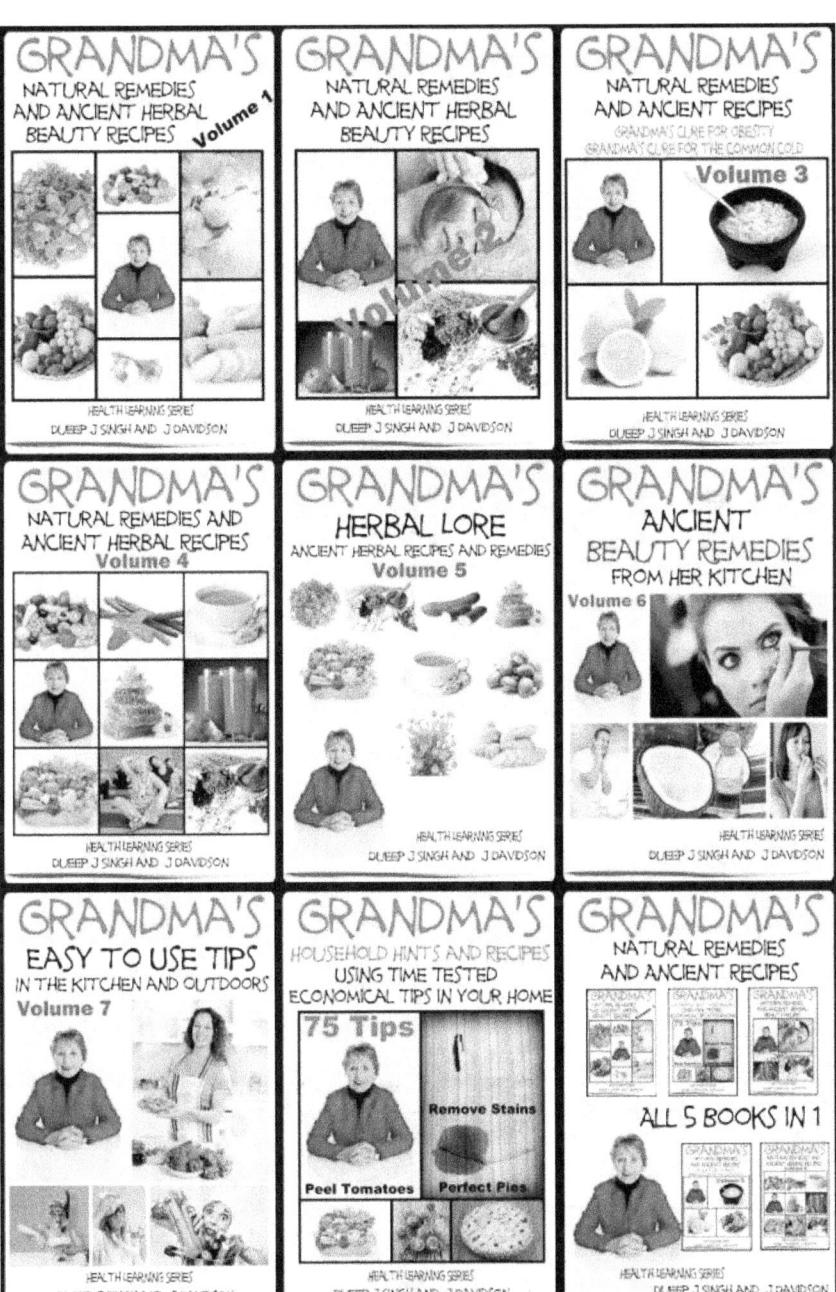

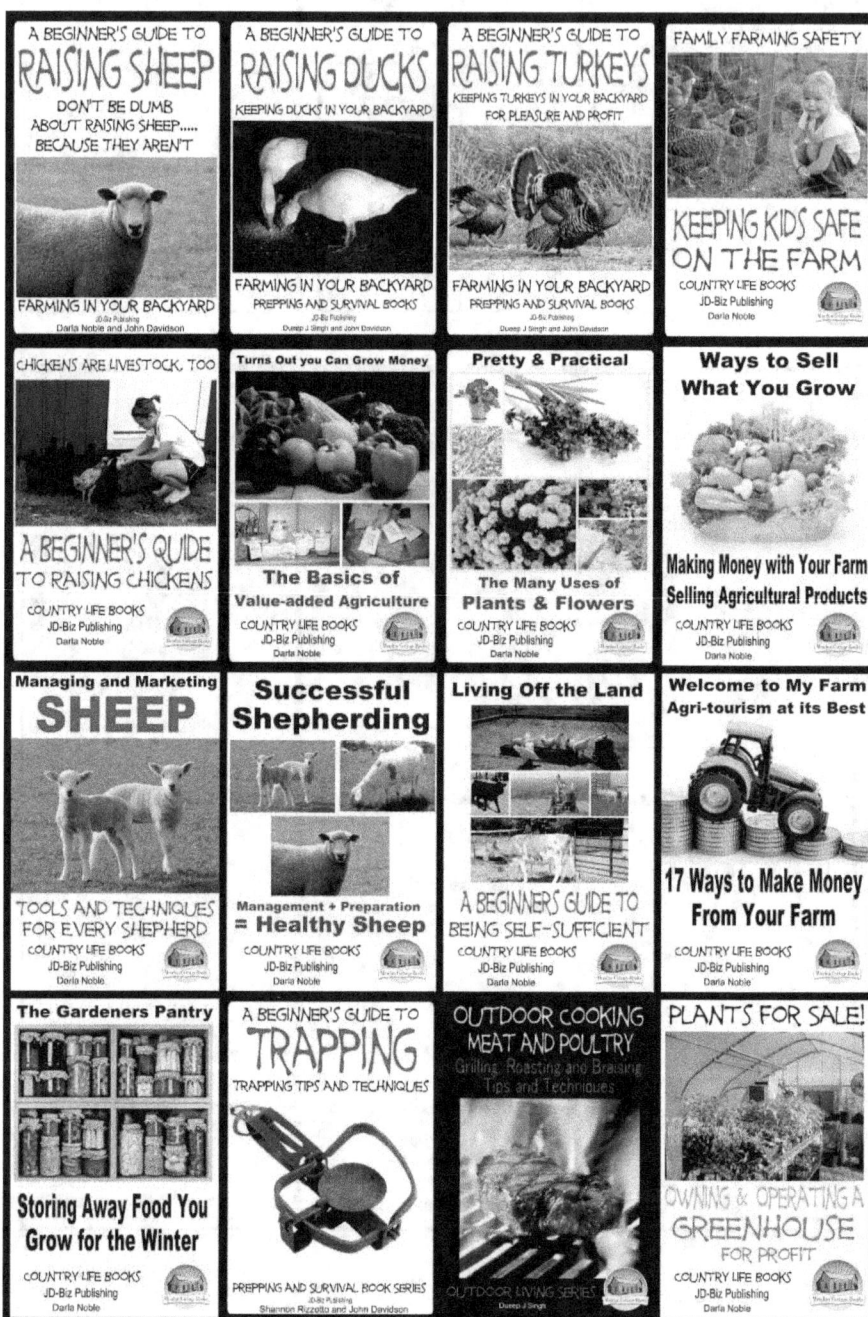

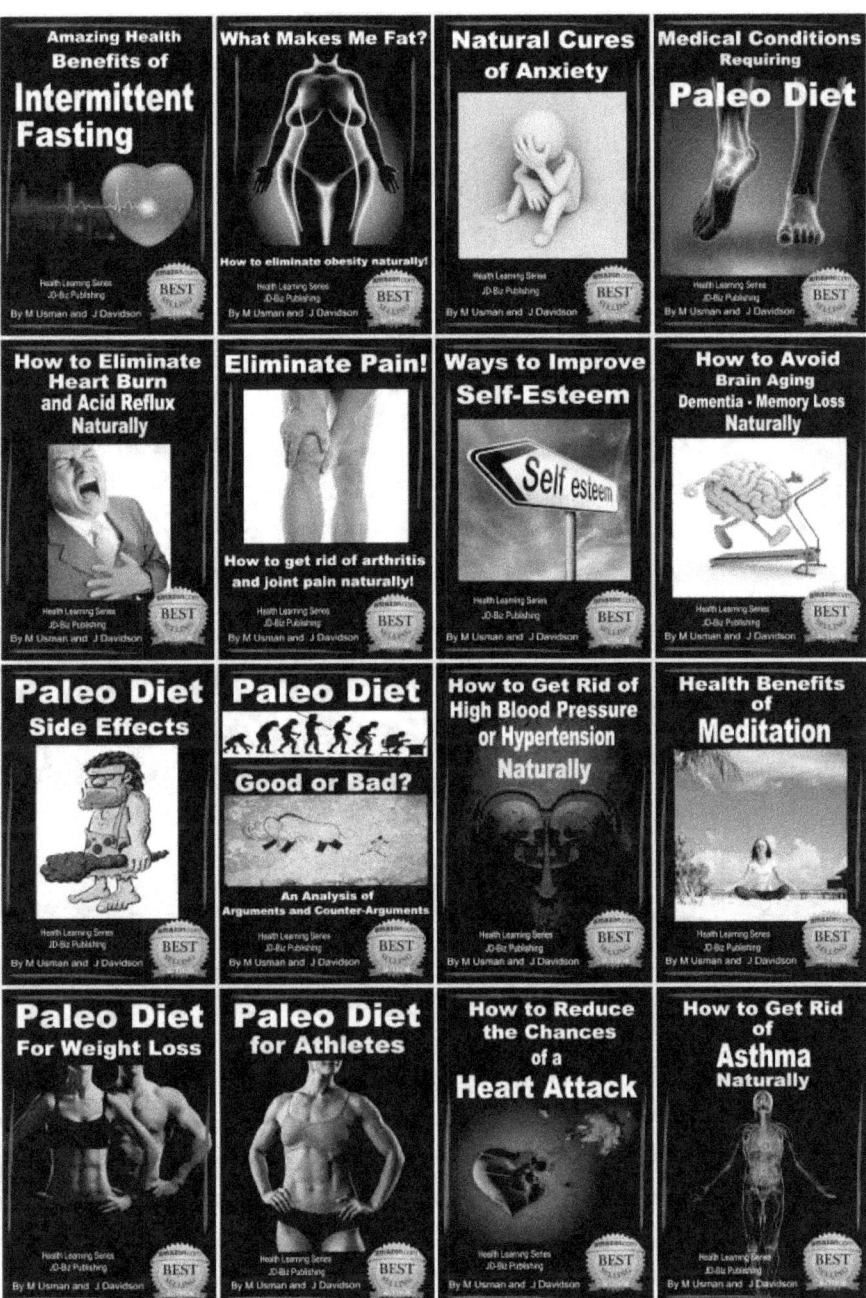

<u>Amazing Animal Book Series</u>

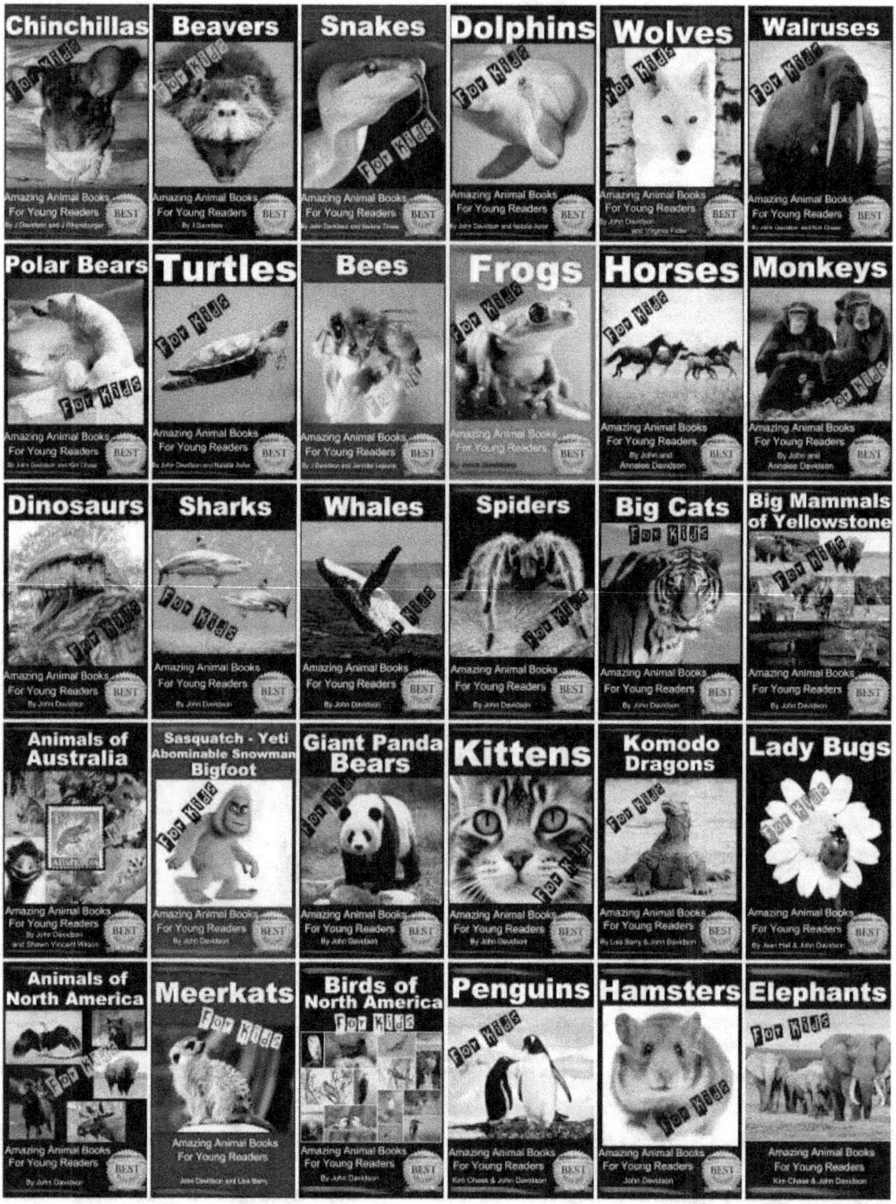

Learn To Draw Series

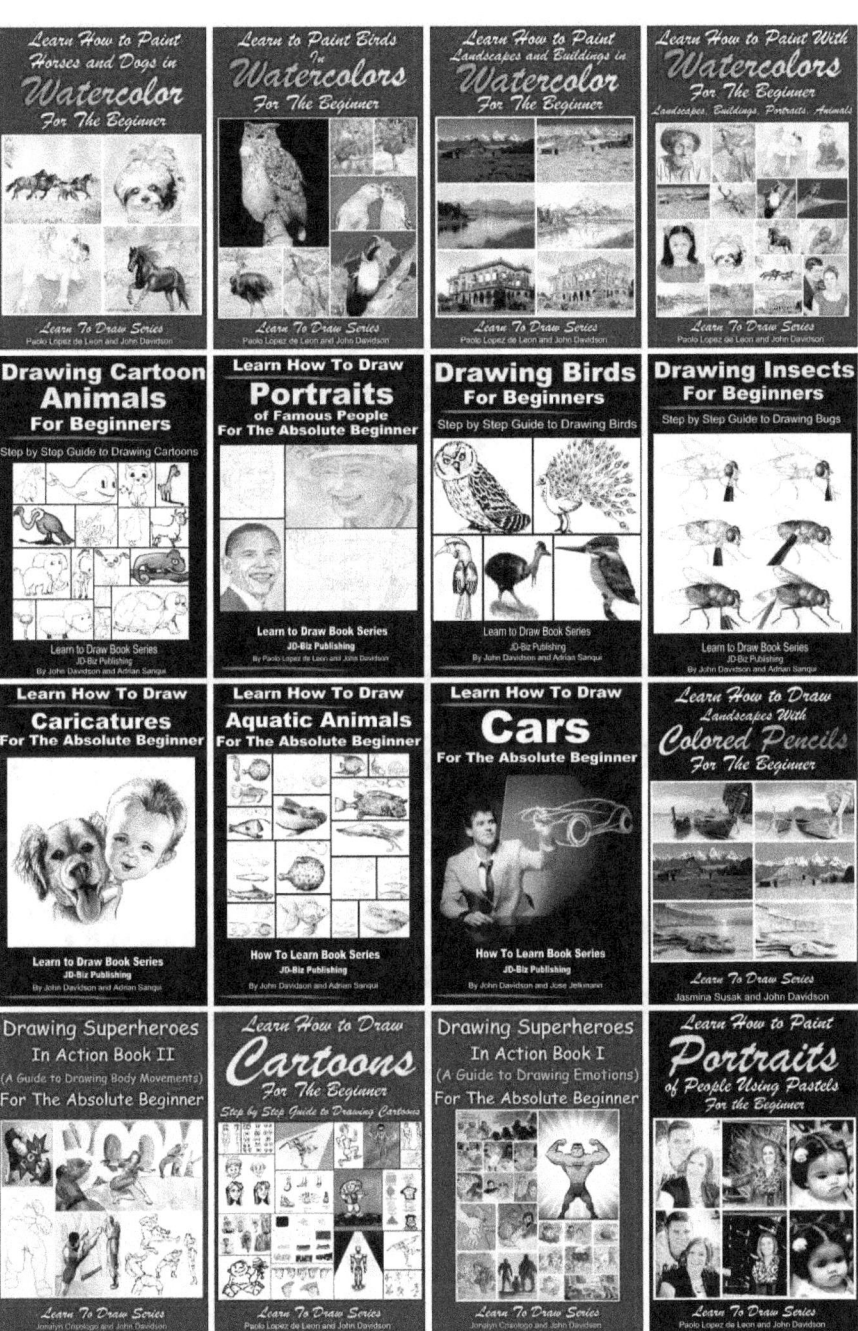

How to Build and Plan Books

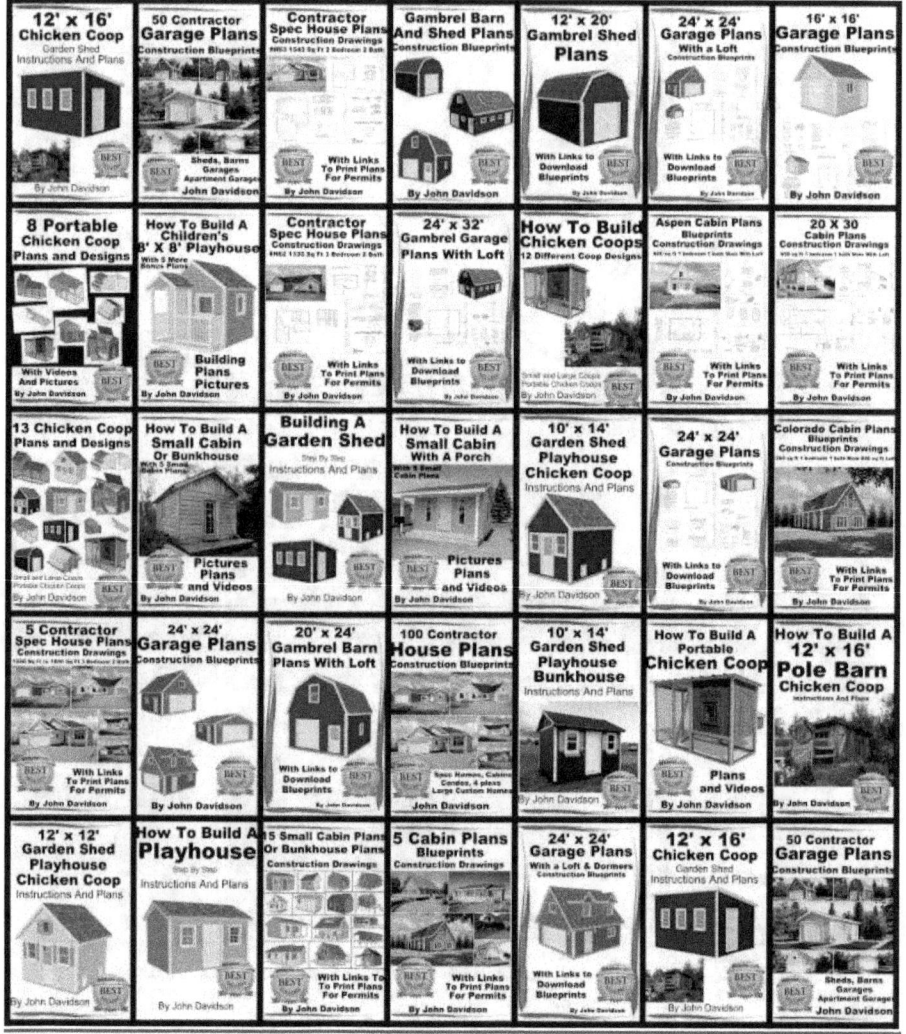

Entrepreneur Book Series

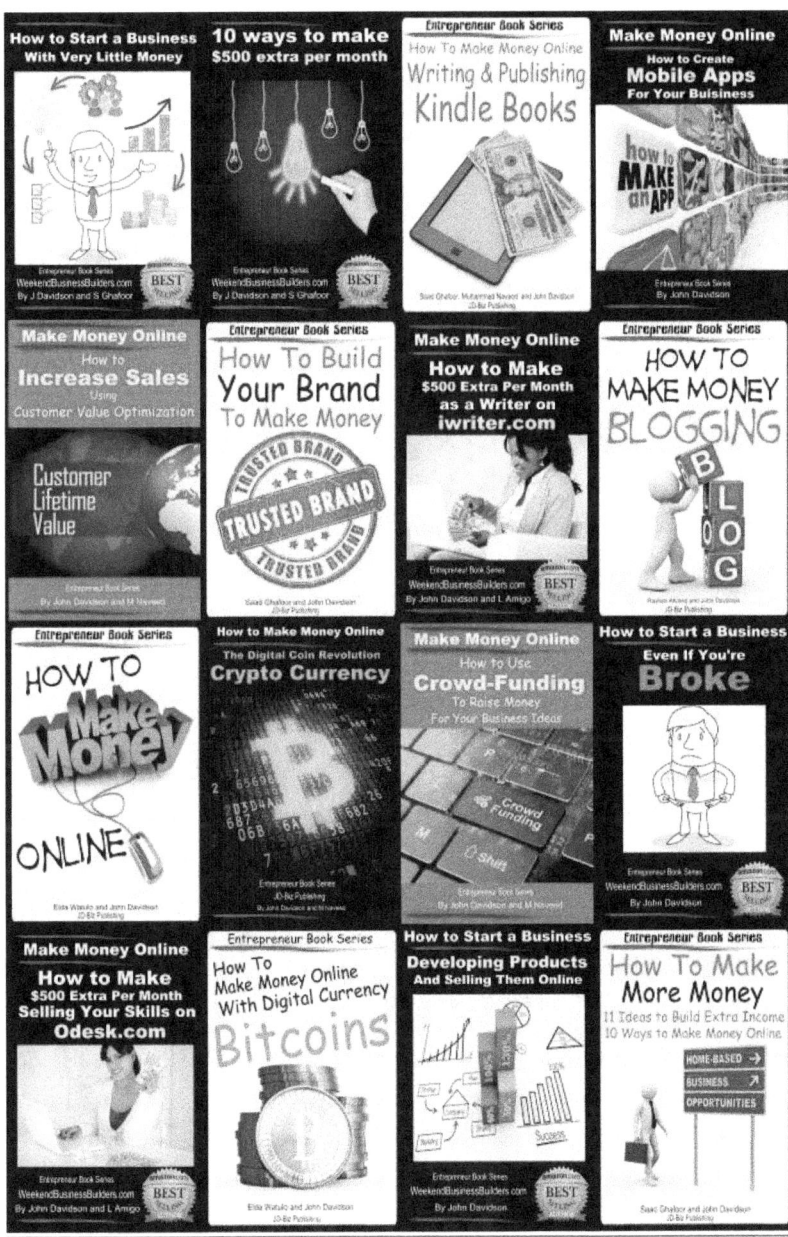

Our books are available at

1. Amazon.com

2. Barnes and Noble

3. Itunes

4. Kobo

5. Smashwords

6. Google Play Books

Publisher

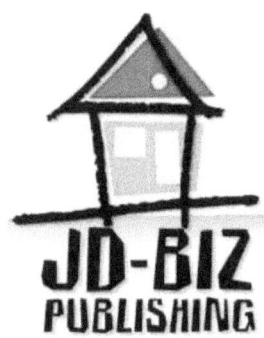

JD-Biz Corp

P O Box 374

Mendon, Utah 84325

http://www.jd-biz.com/

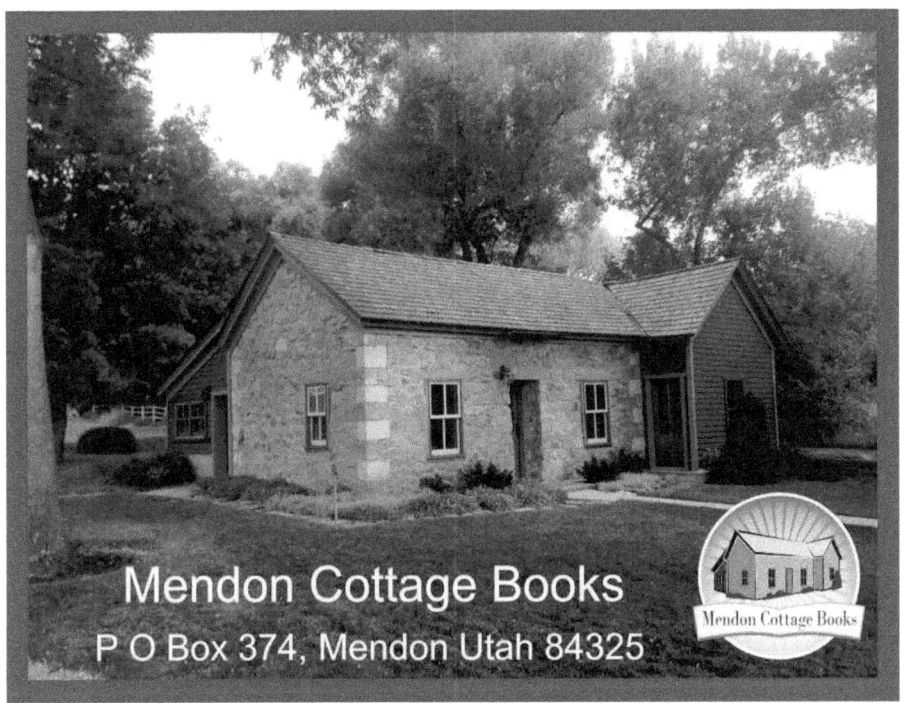

Mendon Cottage Books

P O Box 374, Mendon Utah 84325

www.ingramcontent.com/pod-product-compliance
Lightning Source LLC
Chambersburg PA
CBHW070341290526
45791CB00003B/1424